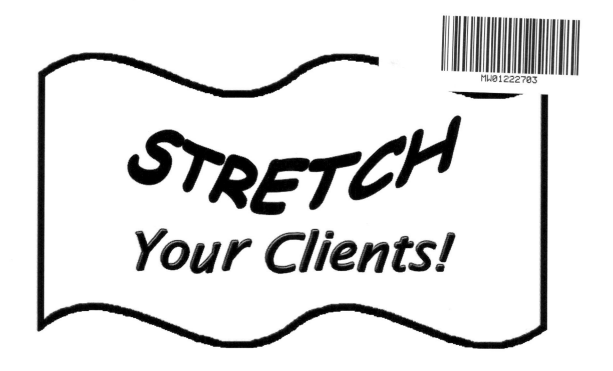

The Bodyworker's Guide to Client Table Stretches

Peggy Lamb, MA, LMT, NCTMB

©2000 Peggy Lamb/Massage Publications. Fourth Edition ©2012. All rights reserved. No part of this publication may be reproduced in any form (including photocopying or storing in any medium by electronic means) without the express written permission of the author.

Additional copies of this book may be obtained from:
www.massagepublications.com

or

Massage Publications
8400 Jamestown Dr #118
Austin, TX 78758

(512) 833-0179

or email

info@massagepublications.com

Disclaimer: This manual is for educational purposes only and should not be considered a substitute for proper training. It is sold with the understanding that the author and publisher are not engaged in rendering medical or other professional services. If medical advice or other expert assistance is required, the services of an appropriate professional should be sought. Information in this book should not be used to diagnose, treat, or prescribe. The author and publisher shall not be held liable for any damages in connection with, or arising out of anyone's interpretation or application of the information in this manual. The practitioner is encouraged to always use sound clinical judgment in making decisions about her/his ability to help each individual and to refer to a qualified professional when the need arises.
© Peggy Lamb (2000-2012)

Photographs by Carol Waid, Grant Gurley, Doug Jopling, Jim Garron and Kelly Page
Models: Nicki Dillon Gurley, Tari Hood, Mary Reynolds and Suzanne Dulany

Acknowledgments

Many people helped me with the writing of this manual. I am fortunate to have numerous supportive friends, colleagues, students and clients. Thanks to my models for being so beautiful and patient; my photographers for their care and professionalism; Wellness Skills, Inc and Texas Healing Arts for providing the space; Grant Gurley, Jeanne Marsh and Martha Hall for editing and proof reading; Laurie Kennerly, Barbara Tanner, Kimberly Howell, Richard Nottingham, Kelly Page, Tim Gurley, David Landsberg and Annie Cooper for their valuable feedback; Ken Duncan for his invaluable help with the layout; Whitney Lowe and Diana Thompson for their generous responses to my many questions and Doug Jopling for the title. This book is dedicated to all of my students from whom I have learned so much.

Peggy Lamb
Austin, Texas
February 2012

TABLE OF CONTENTS

INTRODUCTION	1
THE LONG AND THE SHORT OF STRETCHING	2
GENERAL GUIDELINES FOR STRETCHING	6
POST-INJURY STRETCHING	8
THERAPIST'S BODY MECHANICS	9
NECK & JAW STRETCHES	10
LOW BACK & HIP STRETCHES	17
SHOULDER STRETCHES	32
CHEST & ABDOMINAL STRETCHES	39
HUMERUS & FOREARM STRETCHES	45
THIGH & CALF STRETCHES	50
GLOSSARY	57
SUGGESTED READING	58

STRETCH YOUR CLIENTS!

THE BODYWORKER'S GUIDE TO CLIENT TABLE STRETCHES

INTRODUCTION

This book is designed to be an easy-to-use manual of table stretches that massage therapists can do for and with their clients. During my career as a teacher of various soft tissue techniques I've noticed that both students and practicing massage therapists are uncertain about the role of stretching in bodywork and exactly what stretches to do for specific muscles. Stretching is a crucial ingredient in the maintenance of healthy muscles and in the recovery from a soft tissue injury. I have found that so much time is spent on the strokes (petrissage, friction, etc.), both in the classroom and in a session, that the stretching component is frequently left out or rushed through. I have been guilty of this at times and always regret it.

This manual is not meant to be a comprehensive study about stretching. The stretches shown in the photographs are *not* the only ways to stretch a particular muscle or muscle group. I hope that the reader finds it a concise and practical reference manual and is stimulated to do further reading and research on the subject *(see the suggested reading section.)*

The stretches in this manual are divided into the following sections: **Neck & Jaw**; **Lower Back and Hips**; **Shoulder**; **Chest & Abdominals**; **Humerus & Forearms**; **Thigh & Calf**. The stretches marked with a ★ indicate unassisted self-stretches clients should be encouraged to do on their own. The arrows in some of the photographs refer to the direction of force applied by the therapist. For the sake of clarity most of the stretches are shown without a drape. However, most of the stretches can be done with a drape; just use your creativity. For those stretches in which the draping is too cumbersome, such as a piriformis or iliopsoas stretch, have your client wear gym shorts or have them get dressed and then do the stretch. Some of the stretches can be integrated into a relaxation massage and some are for more specialized bodywork sessions.

Stretching adds an element of expansion into a bodywork session. When we're stretched we feel longer, wider, more alive. We breathe deeper and feel like a million bucks. So, go forth and stretch your clients and yourself!

THE LONG AND THE SHORT OF STRETCHING

WHAT IS STRETCHING?

Stretching is doing the *opposite* of the muscle's action. For example the **supraspinatus** abducts the humerus; in order to stretch the **supraspinatus** you must adduct the humerus. Or for a dual action muscle like the **hamstrings** which bend (flex) the knee and extend the hip you must straighten (extend) the knee and flex the hip. Of course, if you simply straighten the knee and flex the hip or adduct the humerus most people would not feel a stretch. You must take the muscle beyond the natural end point of the range of motion into the *stretch zone*. The stretch zone is the first physiological barrier (first barrier) you meet and it's different for everyone. A quality of a good "stretcher" is a sensitivity for that first barrier; honoring the tissue's boundary by not charging past it but also not stopping before you meet it.

Stretching has its place in a general, feel-good Swedish massage because it helps to *maintain* flexibility. Muscles love to be stretched and massage is the perfect opportunity to stretch them. During massage, the muscles are warm (engorged with blood) and are receptive to stretching. Stretching is important in injury prevention and recovery. When a muscle is torn and injured, its resting length usually shortens. To help our clients recover from an injury, we must know *how* to precisely stretch the targeted muscle.

PHYSIOLOGY OF STRETCHING

Stretching starts in the sarcomere, the basic structural unit of a muscle. The sarcomere contains those famous myofibrils, actin and myosin. When a muscle is stretched, the area of overlap between the myofibrils decreases, allowing the muscle fibers to elongate. The muscle fibers are pulled to their full length, sarcomere by sarcomere. Additional stretching takes place in the surrounding connective tissue. The muscle and collagen fibers align themselves along the same line of force as the stretch. This helps to realign disorganized fibers (both muscle and connective tissue fibers) and contributes to rehabilitating scar tissue.

WHY STRETCH?

The purpose of stretching is to **increase the resting length of a shortened muscle or to maintain an existing healthy resting length**. It improves range of motion and enhances joint function. Muscles contract best from a healthy resting length or slightly longer. Range of motion is much more than biomechanical - it encompasses our body, mind and emotions. When our muscles have healthy resting lengths we have more emotional, spiritual and mental resources to draw upon.

Let's consider a client that is swaybacked (excessive lordosis.) The resting length of that person's **lower erector spinae** is shorter than is optimal, or *locked short*, which means that those muscles are subject to injury. If that person had to suddenly bend over, those muscles would be stretched beyond their capacity and be injured, and the stretch reflex would be activated *(see the stretch reflex section.)*

Many injuries are from overstretching, i.e., the resting length of the muscle was too short to handle the stretch load put on it. When a muscle is injured it can spasm, which is a protective, concentric shortening of the muscle. Left untreated, the muscle can develop scar tissue and a shortened resting length. Massage and guided stretching can reduce and reverse this phenomenon. I love to snow ski and many times I've had my skis separate so I end up doing a split! My adductors have a healthy resting length so they have been able to withstand a sudden yanking stretch and so far I've been able to go on skiing and not have to call the ski patrol.

Another common cause of injured muscles is a phenomenon called *eccentric overloading*. An example of this would be a person who habitually slumps forward so that their thoracic spine is held in a small degree of flexion. This person's thoracic erector spinae are being held in an eccentric contraction or *locked long*. This phenomenon is known as *check-reining*, which means that these muscles are preventing that person from falling over from the force of gravity. In this situation these muscles benefit more from range of motion and strengthening exercises rather than stretching. Locked long tissue still needs flushing and deep tissue work. Because of the tremendous load it's under, locked long tissue often is the first to report pain. When exploring a client's pain pattern, I always ask myself the question, "I wonder if this a locked long pain pattern?" For example, if your client habitually tilts her head to the right, the left scalenes would be locked long and the right scalenes locked short. Both sides need flushing and deep tissue work but only the right scalenes should be stretched. Common locked long tissue on most people include, but are certainly not limited to, the middle and lower traps, the rhomboids, and infraspinatus/teres minor.

THE STRETCH REFLEX

The stretch reflex is a neuromuscular reaction that involves an involuntary contraction, or spasm, of a muscle subjected to a pulling force. It is governed by muscle spindles located throughout the muscle. The spindle is a wonderful hybrid tissue made up of nerve tissue and muscle tissue; nerve for its ability to sense and communicate and muscle for its ability to move.

The function of the stretch reflex is to maintain equilibrium and protect joints. A stretch that is performed too rapidly or too forcefully or is taken too far will activate the stretch reflex. It's crucial that massage therapists understand and watch for the stretch reflex. Stretching should be done **slowly**, **gradually**, **gently** and only ***after*** the muscles have been warmed up. ***Stretching is not a warm-up.***

There may come a time when you inadvertently overstretch a muscle and cause it to spasm while performing a stretch on a client. It happens to the best of us! There are two strategies which are marvelous for counteracting a spasm.

1. Position the joint so that the muscle is put into a passive, concentric contraction. After all, this is what the spasm is doing, bringing the two attachments closer together to prevent further movement and injury. We're just playing a little reverse psychology with the muscle. For example, once I was stretching a client's left **levator scapula** by forward flexing and rotating the neck to the right. I stretched it too far and it spasmed. I immediately returned the head to the table, elevated the client's left shoulder and slightly rotated the neck to the left, replicating the actions of the **levator scapula,** until the spasm cleared. This technique is known by various names including OrthoBionomy and Strain-Counterstrain.

2. Contract the antagonist with an active resisted movement. This strategy makes use of *Reciprocal Inhibition* which governs all paired muscles, agonists/antagonists. When one shortens, the other one has to slightly lengthen in order for movement to occur. By loading the antagonist of the muscle in spasm, it forces the spasm to release. For example, you accidently overstretch a client's **hamstrings** and she yelps in pain. You can save the day by positioning the leg so you can add pressure below the knee and ask them to straighten or extend the knee while you resist her effort. This will shorten the **quadriceps**, thereby stimulating Reciprocal Inhibition. You must add enough resistance so that the number of quadricep fibers recruited matches the number of hamstring fibers that are in spasm.

TYPES OF STRETCHING

1. Passive stretching: the most common form in massage. The client does not assist the therapist except with verbal feedback.

2. Active stretching: the client stretches the muscle with no assistance from the therapist.

3. Active resistive stretches: there are two commonly used types of active resistive stretching: Antagonist-Contract and Agonist-Contract. These techniques are also known as PNF (Proprioceptive Neuromuscular Facilitation) stretches and MET (Muscle Energy Techniques.)

    1. Antagonist-Contract: because of neuromuscular phenomenon known as Reciprocal Inhibition, when the antagonist of the muscle to be stretched is contracted first, the muscle to be stretched (the agonist) will stretch farther than previously had been possible. I call this *priming the stretch pump* and you can do this with any stretch. It's an efficient and easy way to prepare the muscle for stretching. For example, to use this technique on the **quadriceps**, direct the client to bend her knee against resistance, which will contract the **hamstrings**

(the antagonist) and give a signal to the **quadriceps** (the agonist) to release. Hold the contraction for 7-10 seconds, then relax for 2-3 seconds. Then stretch the **quadriceps** by bending the knee and bringing the heel towards the sit bone *(see the section on stretching the thigh for more specific directions.)*

If you're having a problem getting a muscle to stretch, the problem could be in the antagonist. You see this often with subscapularis and pec major because their antagonists, infraspinatus and teres minor are usually locked long. A useful strategy is to warm up the antagonist and do an antagonist contract before stretching the muscle.

2. Agonist-Contract: This technique uses resisted isometric contractions on a stretched muscle to train the stretch receptors to accommodate a greater resting length. The resisted contraction causes a surprising neuromuscular phenomenon that allows the muscle to stretch farther than before. It may seem odd that contracting a muscle helps to stretch it, but it works!

To use this technique on our friend the **quadriceps**, stretch the **quadriceps** by bending the knee and bringing the heel towards the sit bone *(see the section on stretching the thigh for more specific directions.)* When you reach the end point of the stretch, ask the client to contract her **quadriceps** by extending her knee while you provide resistance. I usually ask them to use about ten percent of their effort depending on the size of the client. Have your client hold the contraction for 7-10 seconds, then relax for 2-3 seconds, then stretch the muscle again. Hold the passive stretch for 10-20 seconds. Relax the muscle for 20 seconds and repeat the resisted contraction and then re-stretch. You can do this 3-4 times depending on the client.

Antagonist-Contract and Agonist-Contract are especially useful for clients recovering from an injury or any muscle with an especially short resting length. Any of the stretches in this manual can be done using these two techniques alone or in combination.

GENERAL GUIDELINES FOR STRETCHING

1. Stretch **after** you have massaged the muscle to be stretched. Muscles need to be warm in order to stretch properly and massaging them creates a durable hyperemia. Stretching cold muscles is like stretching a dry sponge.

2. Assess the resting length of the muscle before you stretch it.

3. Ask your client to give you verbal feedback about the stretching. This is crucial to avoid activating the stretch reflex. First ask them where is she feeling the stretch. The stretch should be felt in the muscle that's being stretched or in what I call the "neighborhood association". For example, if you are stretching pectoralis major which is an internal rotator of the humerus, it makes sense that your client may also feel it in latissimus dorsi/teres major which are also internal rotators of the humerus. But, if she is feeling it in the back of the shoulder or upper arm, then you'll need to modify the stretch and calibrate it so you are stretching the correct tissue. Another example would be if you are stretching the iliopsoas. Your client could feel that stretch in any of the nine thigh flexors or even in the abdominal muscles. She should not feel it in the low back. That's a red flag that something is wrong, usually a stabilization issue that can be resolved with a prop.

    After you're certain that your client is feeling the stretch where she should, ask them a good open-ended question like, *"Is there any way I can make this stretch better for you?"* An open-ended question invites more of a truthful response rather than a question like, "Is this ok?"

4. Gently traction the joint before and during the stretch. This aids in maintaining length in the joint and avoiding compression. Experiment with changing the angles of the stretches which will stretch different fibers of the muscles(s).

5. Take the muscle(s) slightly beyond the natural end point of the range of motion into the *"stretch zone"*. This end point is called the physiological barrier. Hold the stretch for a minimum of **15 seconds (3-4 deep breaths)**, encouraging the client to "breathe into" the stretch. After you have held the stretch for 15 seconds see if the muscle will comfortably respond to an additional stretch. Maximum benefit is reached at about 90 seconds. Again, encourage your client to tell you if you're going too far or not far enough. If your client's tissue is fighting the stretch, it's usually because the resting length is so short and the stretch reflex is being engaged. Antagonist and agonist contract are great strategies for reducing the signaling of the stretch reflex. You can also try using a 2-3 second stretch with more repetitions.

6. You can do two or three repetitions of the stretch as needed.

7. The sensation of stretch should be felt in the belly of the muscle and not in the tendon. Muscle fibers have elastic qualities, unlike tendons. For example, in a **hamstrings** stretch, the client should feel the stretch in the center of the **hamstrings** and not near the knee or the ischial tuberosity. This is easier to feel in some muscles, (e.g., hamstrings), than others.

8. Stretching should be slow, gentle, steady and pleasurable. If a person is not used to stretching she may find it uncomfortable at first simply because it's a new sensation. Sometimes a client will confuse a stretching sensation with pain because her experience with movement and stretching techniques is limited. Ask your client to describe the sensation. **As a general rule, if the stretch is causing even moderate pain it should be modified or discontinued. If your client is recovering from an injury, work within her pain threshold.**

9. Contraindications: absolute contraindications are an injury in the acute stage, joint hyper-flexibility and muscles that are over-stretched/locked long. Approach other contraindications on a case-to-case basis. My rule of thumb is, "when in doubt, leave it out," till I consult a physical therapist. *"Let pain be your guide!"*

10. Know the actions and attachments of the muscle you are stretching. A strong foundational knowledge of anatomy is indispensable for intelligent, intuitive bodywork.

POST-INJURY STRETCHING

The same guidelines apply to a client recovering from an injury. In addition to the points mentioned above, there are several other factors to consider:

1. *Is the injury acute, sub-acute, or chronic?* Stretching is contraindicated in the acute stage of any injury.

2. *Is this a first-, second- or third-degree muscle strain?* A first-degree muscle strain involves only a few muscle fibers with mild inflammation and rapid recovery. A second-degree muscle strain involves more fibers and possibly the tendon, with moderate inflammation. A third-degree muscle strain involves over half of the muscle's fibers and its tendons, with severe inflammation and pain. Only first- and second-degree strain should be treated with massage, and it is recommended to have physician approval before treating a second-degree strain.

3. *Severity of the injury.* The more severe the injury, the slower you have to go. You may want to spend the first few sessions doing only massage, then gradually include gentle range of motion exercises over the next few sessions and finally building up to gentle passive stretches.

4. *Client psychology.* People who have had a long-term chronic injury may be depressed. Depression intensifies pain and lowers pain thresholds. This client may not be motivated to continue her exercise program. She may just want to get the "feel-good" massage and not be stretched. Don't push the client, but explain the importance of stretching for a full recovery.

5. *At-home stretching.* This is for everyone, but especially for the client recovering from an injury. Remind your clients that muscle health and recovery is a duet, not a solo, and that the client's participation is crucial.

Buy a book on self-stretching and make sure the client knows how to do the stretches. I suggest spending the last five minutes of a session reviewing the self-stretches for the client's homework. Remember, the stretches marked with a **star** ★ indicate unassisted self-stretches clients should be encouraged to do on their own.

THERAPIST'S BODY MECHANICS

The importance of using good body mechanics when stretching a client cannot be overstated. Use this simple rule of thumb: ***If it hurts you, don't do it, or adapt the stretch so it's comfortable for you.*** Here are some tips:

- Keep your three body weights (head, torso, and pelvis) in alignment.

- Keep your head in alignment with your spine: avoid being *"visually enthralled"* (lowering your head to peer down). (Credit to Bob King, past president of the AMTA, for coining that wonderful term!).

- The 3 L's: Leaning, Lunging and Leverage – lean into your lunges and use your body weight as leverage to lift your client's body parts. (Again, credit to Bob King for coining the term "The 3 L's".)

- Keep your feet facing the direction of your movement and the force you are applying.

- Center of gravity or hara: move from this core point (two inches below navel) and allow the pelvis to be in a neutral (neither swaybacked nor tucked under) position. I like to imagine a flashlight attached to my belly button so the light can lead my movement.

- Maintain a broad, level base of support: use the feet and legs to support you.

- Keep the scapulae and shoulder joints in a neutral position: avoid holding the scapulae in a protracted (abducted) position and internally rotating the shoulder joints while you work.

- Let the shoulder girdle hang like a yoke: this helps to keep the torso upright and sitting on the pelvis. Our tendency is either to collapse at the sternum or to raise the sternum and the shoulders too high.

- Keep the wrists and elbows in neutral position: avoid, when possible, hyperextension of the wrist which over-stretches the flexor group, and, work with a straight (not locked) elbow when possible.

- Soft knees: keep the knees gently flexed and use them as levers to raise and lower your body.

NECK & JAW

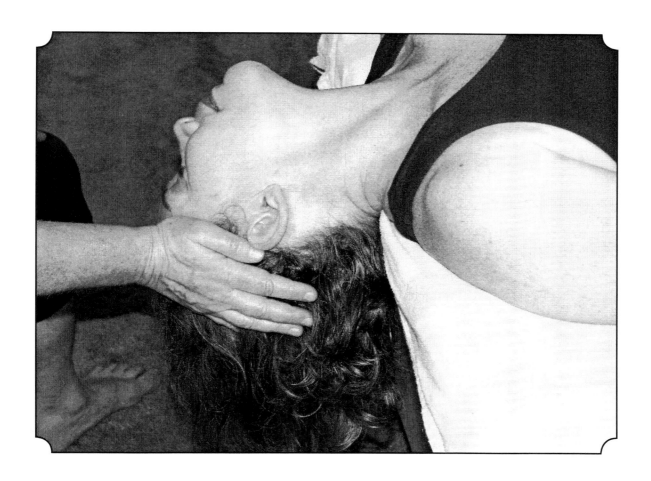

STRETCHES

MUSCLE ACTIONS

Muscle actions vary depending on where the body is positioned in space and how gravity is acting on it. The actions listed in this book are the generally accepted actions of each muscle. There are many excellent books with more detailed information and kinesiology. A personal favorite is Dr. Janet Travell's and Dr. David Simons: "Myofascial Pain and Dysfunction: The Trigger Point Manual".

NECK AND JAW

Levator scapula: elevates the scapula and rotates the neck to the same side; downward rotation of the scapula.

Splenius capitis and cervicis: extends and rotates the head and neck to the same side.

Scalenes: forward and laterally flexes the neck, stabilizes the neck and assists in inspiration.

Semispinalis: extends the neck and head.

Sternocleidomastoid: stabilizes the neck; forward and laterally flexes the neck; rotates the neck to the opposite side.

Sub-occipitals: rocks, tilts, rotates, and extends the head.

Trapezius (upper fibers): laterally flexes the neck, assists in rotating the neck to the opposite side; elevates the shoulders, upwardly rotates the scapula.

Masseter and Temporalis: elevates (closes) and retracts the mandible.

1. LEVATOR SCAPULAE, MULTIFIDI, SEMISPINALIS, SPELENIUS CAPITIS AND CERVICIS, UPPER TRAPEZIUS, SUPERIOR FIBERS OF ERECTOR SPINAE, AND SUB-OCCIPITALS STRETCH:

Client is supine. Gently traction the neck then lift client's head and neck off the

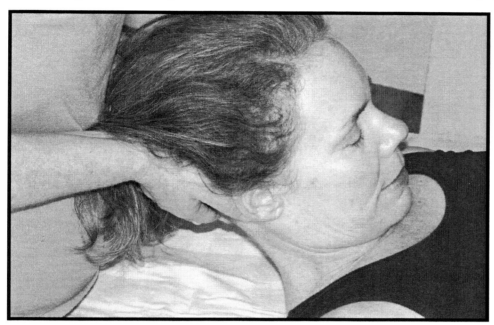

table into forward flexion while maintaining the traction. Keep your hands close together in a cradle hold and your elbows close into your body to reduce strain on your neck and shoulders.

After holding the forward flexion for 15-30 seconds, add varying degrees of rotation to one side, then the other, depending on which side needs the stretch. Combining forward flexion with rotation stretches the neck rotators. For example, to stretch the right **splenius capitis**, **cervicis** and **levator scapula** you would first forward flex the neck then rotate it to the left. To increase the stretch, gently press down on opposite shoulder.

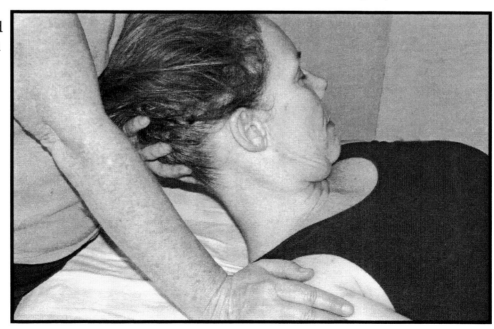

2. SUB-OCCIPITAL STRETCH:

This stretch is especially useful for those clients with a forward head posture. With a forward head, the posterior cervicals are usually overstretched while the sub-occipitals are shortened. In that scenario, you would avoid doing a neck flexion stretch, (shown on previous page), and isolate the sub-occipitals by placing the client in a side-lying position. This stretch can also be done supine and prone. In the supine position just lift the head off the table far enough so your fingers can hook under the occipital ridge - avoid flexing the neck. Since these muscles are locked short on so many of us, I do this stretch in all three positions when working on a client with chronic neck issues.

Have the client tuck her chin into her throat so as to just flex the head and **not** the neck. This provides an antagonist-contract by shortening the deep neck flexors. Place your thumb on one side of the spine, under the occipital ridge, and your fingers on the other side of the spine, also under the occipital ridge. Gently push up towards the top of the head, increasing the head flexion.

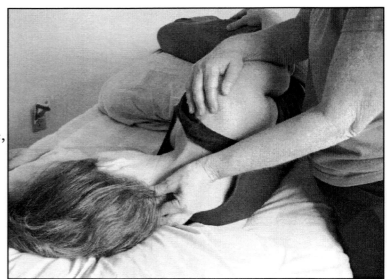

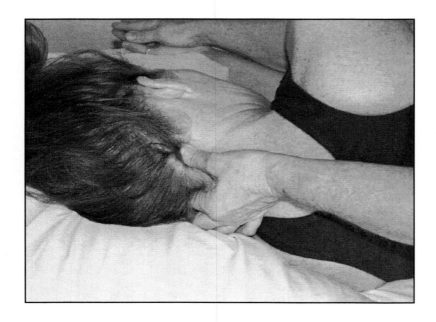

3. SCALENES AND UPPER TRAPEZIUS STRETCH:

The following three photographs illustrate how to stretch the medial, anterior, and posterior scalenes. All three stretch various fibers of the **upper trapezius and the sternocliedomastoid**. Notice in photos B and C that rotation has been added to the primary movement of lateral flexion (side-bending.)

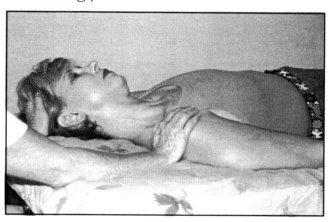

A. Client is supine with the shoulders externally rotated (palms up). Therapist laterally flexes the neck (ear to shoulder). For the **medial scalene**, *(photo right)*, the neck is in pure lateral flexion with no rotation. In the photograph to the right, the therapist's right hand is stabilizing and pressing down on the client's right shoulder while the left hand is gently pressing the head and neck towards the left shoulder. For best results, push from the parietal/occipital area. Remember to maintain traction on the neck.

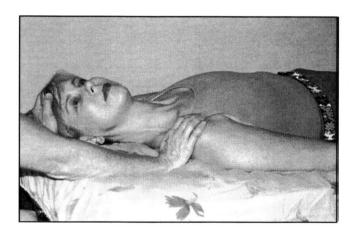

B. To stretch the anterior scalene, *(photo left)*, maintain lateral flexion and ask the client to turn her head towards the side of the neck being stretched (in this case the right side.) I suggest rotating the neck only 20-30 degrees.

C. To stretch the **posterior scalene**, *(photo right)*, maintain lateral flexion and ask the client to turn her head *away* from the side of the neck being stretched (in this case the right side). Again, the degree of rotation should be 20-30 degrees to be specific to posterior scalene. For a **trapezius** stretch, simply increase the degree of rotation.

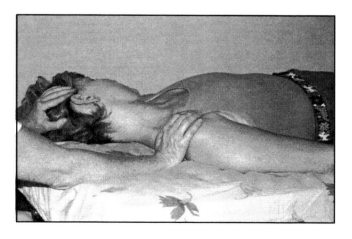

4A. STERNOCLEIDOMASTOID AND SCALENES STRETCH:

Client is supine. Ask your client to scoot her body so the head can come off the table. It's important that the client use her spine, legs and feet to inch back like a worm and not use the neck muscles, which may be her first inclination. Make sure your client's shoulders are on the table and just the neck is off the table. ***This stretch is contraindicated for clients who have disc abnormalities or other cervical dysfunctions or have had neck surgery. You may want to try the alternate stretch on the nest page.***

A. Bilateral stretch. Gently (gravity is doing most of your work!) increase the hyperextension by pressing on the chin or tractioning the ribs and sternum towards the feet *(not shown)* and cranium.

B. Rotate the head 20-30 degrees right and press on the left cranium to stretch the **left** SCM.

C. Rotate the head 20-30 degrees left and press on the right cranium to stretch the **right** SCM.

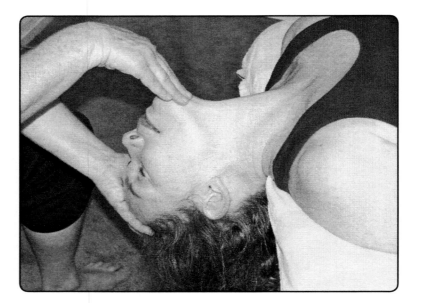

A.

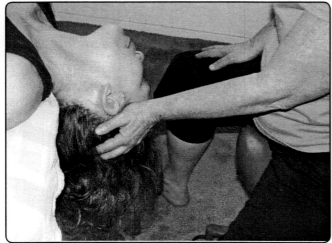

B.

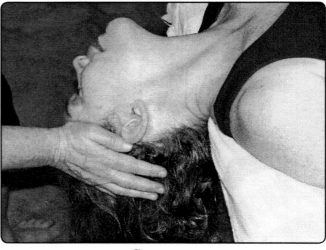

C.

Slowly bring the client's head back to table level and ask the client to scoot her body back onto the table using the legs and feet.

4B. ALTERNATE STRETCH FOR STERNOCLEIDOMASTOID:

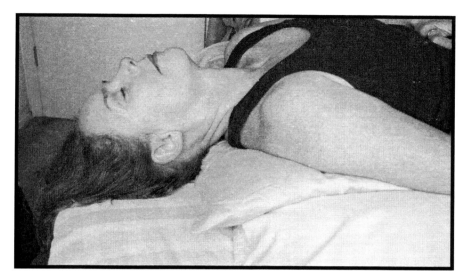

Client is supine. Prop one or two pillows under the client's mid-back, depending on her flexibility, so the head is in hyperextension, yet supported by the table. Proceed with stretch as described above. This position is also great for deepening the breath and stretching the pectoralis major (the arms must be out to the side; see section on the Chest.) You can massage the lower body while the client enjoys this stretch.

JAW STRETCH

1. MASSETER AND TEMPORALIS STRETCH:

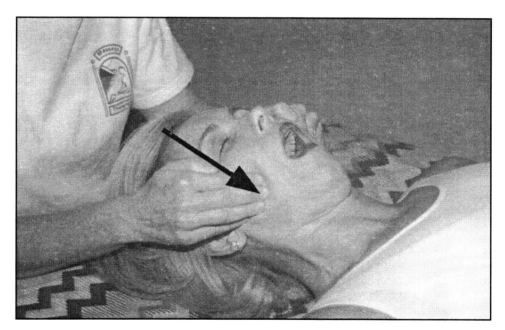

Although the masseter and temporalis are not neck muscles, their tonus impacts the neck and vice versa. Including soft tissue work and stretching of these muscles during your neck sequence is beneficial.
Client is supine. Ask the client to open her mouth as wide as possible without discomfort. Gently push (depress) the jaw down from the tempro-mandibular joint.

LOW BACK & HIP

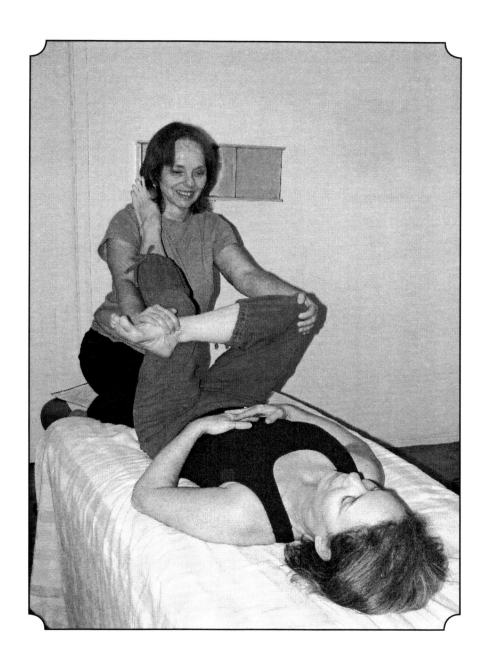

STRETCHES

LOWER BACK AND HIP

Erector Spinae: extends the spine; also contributes to rotation and lateral flexion of the spine.

Gluteus Maximus: extension of the femur at the hip; assists in lateral rotation and helps maintain erect posture.

Gluteus Minimus: abduction and internal rotation of the femur; assists in stabilization of the pelvis during single-limb stance.

Gluteus Medius: abduction and internal rotation of the femur; stabilizes the pelvis during single-limb stance.

Iliopsoas (psoas): flexes the femur at the hip and plays a significant role in maintaining upright posture.

Multifidi: extends and rotates the spine.

Piriformis: external rotator of the femur; assists in stabilizing the pelvis during weight-bearing activities. The piriformis becomes an internal rotator when the femur is flexed and the lower leg crosses the midline.

Quadratus Lumborum: lateral flexor of the spine; elevates (hikes) the same-side hip; contributes to extension and rotation of the spine. Stabilizes the lumbar spine on the pelvis.

Rotatores: extends and rotates the spine.

Tensor fasciae latae: assists in flexion, abduction, and internal rotation of the thigh.

1. LUMBAR PORTION OF ERECTOR SPINAE AND GLUTEUS MAXIMUS STRETCH: ★

Client is supine, therapist is standing on the side of the back to be stretched.

Step 1: Flex thigh to 90 degrees.

Step 2: Traction femur up towards the ceiling and angle the thigh to the outside

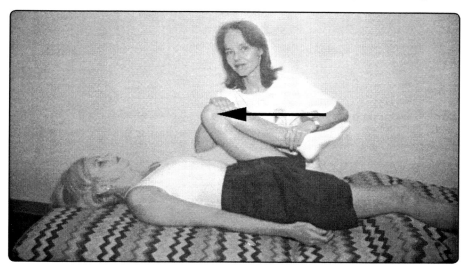

then increase the degree of thigh flexion. This maneuver creates space in the thigh joint which helps eliminate the crimping pain at the thigh joint many people feel with this stretch. This pain/crimping is usually due to short thigh flexors, so if the traction doesn't work, massage the thigh flexors and try again.

Step 3: Increase the thigh flexion and press the leg into the torso. To ensure an erector spinae stretch, push the thigh towards the client's head far enough so that the sit bone comes off the table. If the pelvis stays flat, only the gluteus maximus would be stretched. Experiment with different angles to stretch various fibers of these muscles but always make sure the pelvis is stable.

To stabilize the opposite side and get a gentle *iliopsoas* stretch on the other leg, use your other hand to gently press the extended thigh into the table.

Clients should be instructed to do this as an unassisted self-stretch by hugging one or both knees into the torso.

The stretch on the previous page is easily integrated into a Swedish massage. To perform it with a drape, simply create a "diaper" drape. For extra privacy you can ask the client to hold on to the ends of the drape.

Join this stretch with next two stretches for a fabulous combination your clients will love.

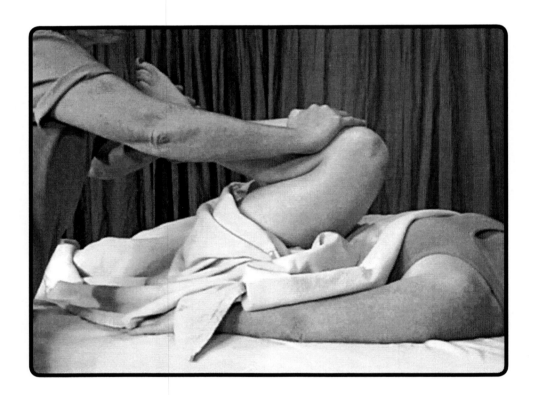

2. LUMBAR PORTION OF ERECTOR SPINAE, MULTIFIDI, ROTATORES AND GLUTEUS MAXIMUS STRETCH: ★

Client is supine.

Step 1: Flex the thigh to 90 degrees or less. With your downhill hand, gently push the client's hip away from you while your uphill hand stabilizes the client's torso by pressing down on the shoulder.

Step 2: Traction the iliac crest toward the feet as you push the hip away from you.

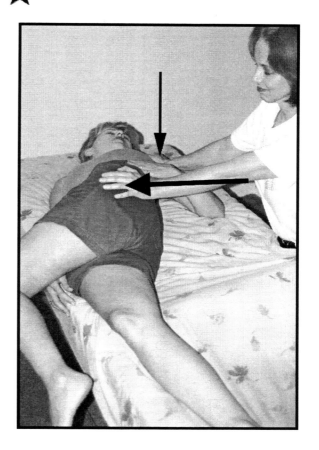

The amount you twist the client's hips depends on their flexibility. As always, solicit feedback from your client. In the photograph to the right, the therapist is standing on the side to be stretched, but this stretch can also be done standing on the opposite side *(shown below.)* If that is more comfortable, simply pull the client's hips towards you with one hand while stabilizing the torso with your other hand. Clients should be instructed to do this as an unassisted self-stretch by guiding the thigh across the body with the opposite arm.

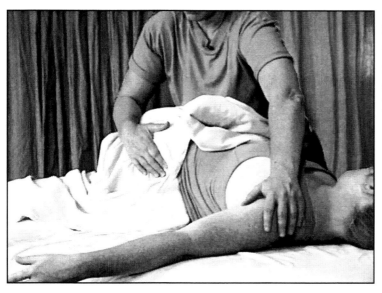

Stretch shown with a drape. Notice that the therapist is stabilizing the torso by pressing on the shoulder, giving a gentle pectoralis major stretch to the client.

{Reminder: Stretch after you have massaged the muscle to be stretched.}

3. LUMBAR PORTION OF THE ERECTOR SPINAE, MULTIFIDI, ROTATORES, GLUTEUS MAXIMUS AND HAMSTRING STRETCH:

I often combine this stretch with the previous two stretches for a dynamic lower back series.

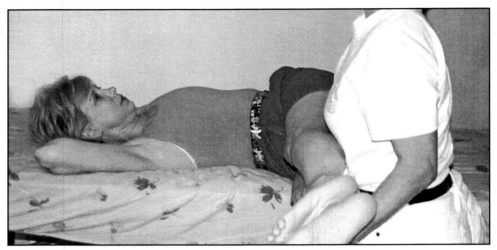

Client is supine. Lift the legs from beneath the ankles and slowly walk the legs around towards the client's head. As you move the clients legs to the side of the table, they will naturally fall on top of one another. Hold for 15-30 seconds, then do the other side. It is important that the torso stays flat; if you see the client's torso twisting, instruct the client to stabilize the torso by holding onto the table. You can have the client bend her knees for a less intense hamstring stretch. Bending the knees moves the stretch more into the low back and hips.

This stretch is one your clients will love and is easily integrated into a Swedish massage. Draping is a cinch - simply take the fitted sheet and wrap the ends around your client's feet *(shown below.)* Voila, you've created a foolproof drape!

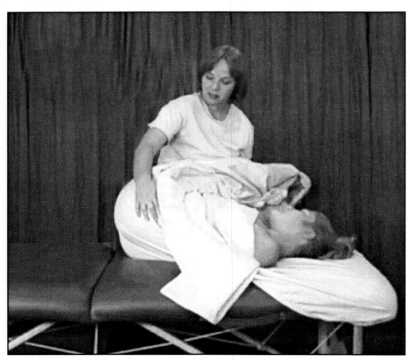

Notice that the therapist's right hand is on the clients pelvis. She's gently tractioning and pressing the hips toward herself to create a variation which intensifies the lower back stretch.

{Reminder: Gently traction the joint before and during the stretch.}

4. ERECTOR SPINAE AND MULTIFIDI (CAT STRETCH):

Client is on hands and knees and is instructed to bring the head and tailbone towards each other while "humping" the mid-back. Place one hand on the lower back and one hand between the scapulae. Using the heel of your hands, traction with a slight downward pressure. Imagine you are separating the vertebrae. Make sure the client's wrists and shoulders are in alignment and the elbows are lengthened. Clients should be instructed to do this as an unassisted self-stretch.

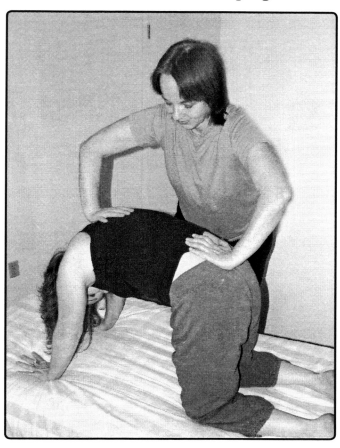

{Reminder: Ask your client to give you verbal feedback about the stretch. This is crucial to avoid activating the stretch reflex. A good open-ended question that invites response is, "Is there any way I can make this stretch better for you?"}

5. LUMBAR PORTION OF THE ERECTOR SPINAE AND MULTIFIDI STRETCH (POSE OF CHILD STRETCH): ★

This stretch is great for people with lordosis. It's easily integrated into a prone back sequence because the drape stays neatly in place as the client gets into position. I like to combine this with the Cat Stretch on the previous page.

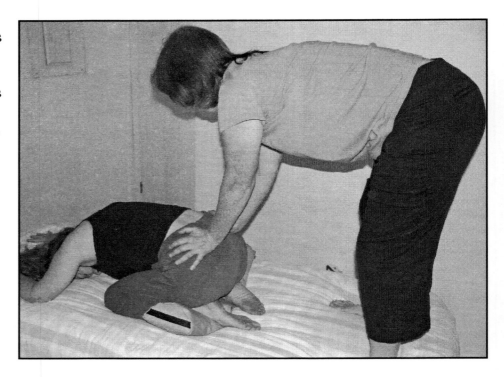

Client kneels, then sits back on her heels with the chest resting on the knees and the arms resting on the table.

Step 1: Place your hands on your client's iliac crests. Traction the pelvis toward you, then press the hips down toward the table.

If the client feels pain in the knees, there's several ways to prop:
1. Have her separate the knees.
2. Place a pillow on the calves to decrease the degree of knee flexion.
If the pain persists, discontinue the stretch.

If the client has a large girth you can place a pillow on the front of the thighs to create space for the belly and diaphragm which allows for easier breathing.

A bolster under the ankles usually resolves any ankle discomfort. For more leverage, you can push from the front or sit on the client *(see next page)*. If you are uncomfortable being on the table, simply have the client get dressed and you can do this stretch on the floor. Clients should be instructed to do this as an unassisted self-stretch.

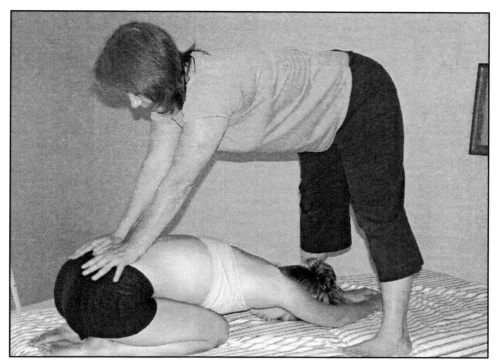

Another fabulous variation of this stretch is to push from the front. Therapists, make sure your spine is straight and your shoulder joints are externally rotated.

The ultimate version of this stretch! Sit sacrum to sacrum, using your sacrum like your hands, as described above.

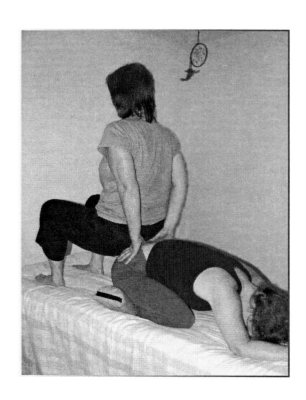

6. TENSOR FASCIAE LATAE; ILIO-TIBIAL BAND; GLUTEUS MINIMUS & MEDIUS (ANTERIOR FIBERS); AND SOME FIBERS OF THE QUADRATUS LUMBORUM STRETCH:

This is a great stretch for runners. Client is supine. Therapist is standing on the **opposite** side of table of the leg being stretched.

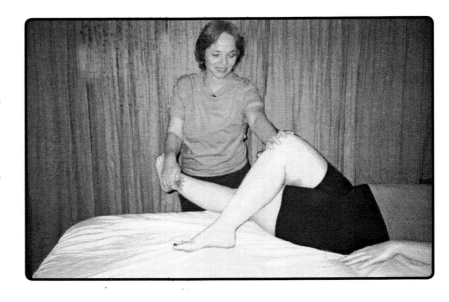

Step 1: Cross the client's legs and place the opposite foot on the outside of the knee of the leg to be stretched. Place one hand on opposite knee to stabilize; make sure to keep that knee in neutral alignment and do **not** internally rotate the femur.

Step 2: Grasp the ankle of the leg to be stretched and slide it across towards you (adduct the leg.)

Make sure the pelvis does not torque or lift and the client does not feel strain in the lower back. I often give my clients the image of a heavy sandbag resting on their pelvis, which helps keep it stable and flat on the table.

You can experiment with externally and internally rotating the femur of the leg being stretched to stretch different fibers of the muscles.

If the client feels pain in the knee, adduct the leg from underneath the knee instead of the ankle as shown below.

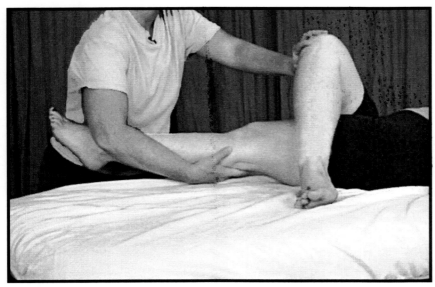

If your client has knee pain try this variation of adducting the leg by lifting from just below the knee.

7. QUADRATUS LUMBORUM, GLUTEUS MINIMUS AND MEDIUS and TENSOR FASCIAE LATAE/ILIO-TIBIAL BAND STRETCH: ★

Client is side-lying on the side opposite to be stretched and moves her body to the edge of the table. Guide the top leg to hang off the edge of the table. The knee needs to clear the table; sometimes it takes a bit of trial and error to achieve this while maintaining the client's alignment. If you're having trouble getting the knee to clear the table, ask her to scoot her upper body away from you and her rear end towards you. Stabilize the pelvis with your body to prevent rotation or over-arching of the lower back. A pillow under the clients' waist can help with positioning and increase the stretch.

Step 1: Gently press down on the femur (less intense) or the calf (more intense) of the leg being stretched with your downhill hand. The client's upper arm must be above the ribs, reaching up towards her head. With your uphill hand traction the iliac crest away from the ribs. Hold for 15-30 seconds.

Step 2: Move your upper hand to the rib case (see below) and traction it away from the pelvis, while **maintaining** the pressure on the femur or calf.

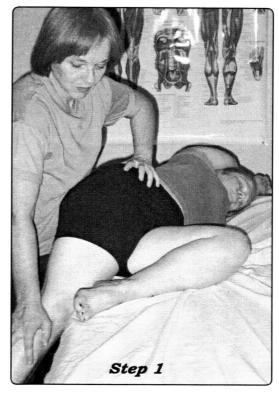
Step 1

Step 3: To come out of the stretch, lift the leg back onto the table, so the client does not engage the muscle.

If letting the leg hang is too painful, arrange a chair for the ankle to rest on for about a minute, then see if the leg can hang without pain. Clients should be instructed to do this as an unassisted self-stretch by letting the leg hang off the edge of a bed.

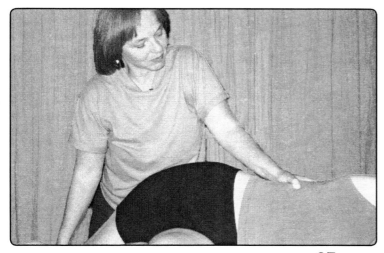

Step 2:
Traction the rib case away from the pelvis.

8. GLUTEUS MINIMUS AND MEDIUS, TENSOR FASCIAE LATAE, AND SOME FIBERS OF THE QUADRATUS LUMBORUM STRETCH:

Client is lying on the side to be stretched, with the lower arm above the ribs. Your uphill hand tractions and stabilizes the pelvis while the downhill arm wraps around both ankles and lifts the lower legs off the table and gently pulls them towards the client's head. The knees and thighs remain on the table.

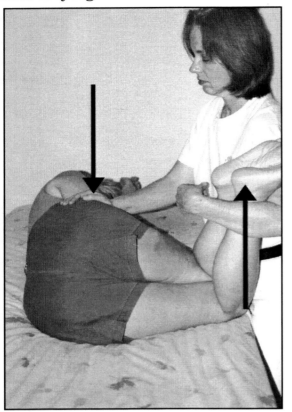

I've found that some clients feel this in their quadratus lumborum more than the preceding stretch while other clients feel very little from this stretch. It's good to know several stretches for a muscle because we're all unique and what works on one client may not work on another.

9. GLUTEUS MINIMUS AND MEDIUS, TENSOR FASCIAE LATAE & ILIIO-TIBIAL BAND STRETCH:

Here's yet another way to stretch the abductors of the femur. If you are short, like me, you'll need to climb on the table.

Client is lying on the side to be stretched. Your uphill hand stabilizes the pelvis while the downhill arm wraps under the client's femur and lifts it off the table towards the ceiling.

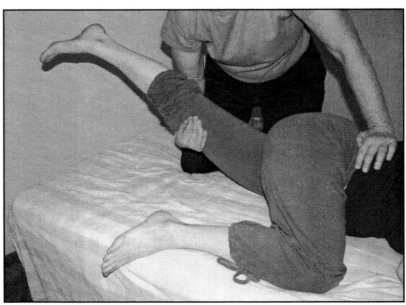

10. PIRIFORMIS STRETCH:

Client is supine.

Step 1: Have the client place the ankle of the leg to be stretched on top of the opposite thigh so that the leg to be stretched is externally rotated. *(The piriformis becomes an internal rotator when the femur is flexed and abducted and the lower leg crosses the midline. This is why we externally rotate the thigh to stretch the piriformis.)*

Step 2: Ask the client to lift the opposite foot off the table, which they can place on your thigh *(as shown in photo A)* or shoulder *(photo B)*, or a bolster depending on the degree of thigh flexion needed. The degree of thigh flexion of the opposite leg determines the intensity of the piriformis stretch. Ask your client exactly where they feel the stretch. If they only feel it in the hip flexors, increase the amount of thigh flexion of the opposite leg.

Step 3: Increase the degree of external rotation by pulling the client's knee toward you and pushing her ankle away from you.

(Note: If you are working with a client who has been suffering from severe piriformis syndrome, be careful with this stretch. Wait until you have worked with the client several times before performing this stretch, and then proceed with caution.

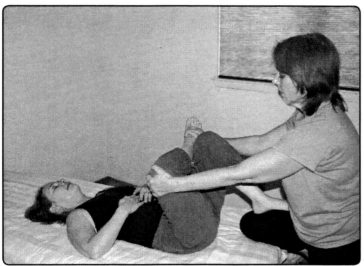

Photo A

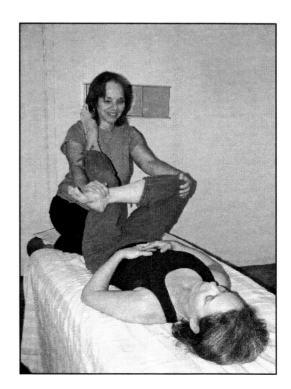

Photo B

11A. ILIOPSOAS AND THIGH FLEXOR STRETCH SUPINE:

Client is supine and has moved to the end of the table as far as possible so the legs can hang freely. Client grasps the opposite knee and hugs it.

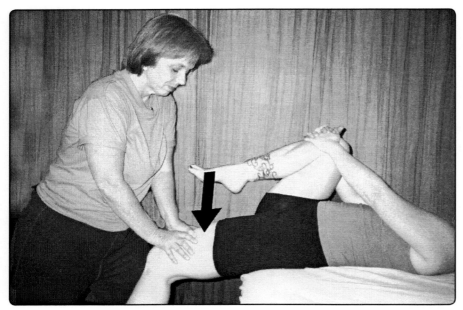

Step 1: Gently traction the femur then press the leg to be stretched towards the floor into hyperextension. This also stretches the secondary thigh flexors: ***rectus femoris, tensor fascia latae, sartorius, pectineus, gracilis, adductors longus, brevis and magnus***.

Step 2: Hold for 15-30 seconds.

Step 3: Experiment with rotating the femur internally and externally to stretch different fibers of these muscles.
Step 4: To come out of the stretch, lift the leg back onto the table, so the client does not engage the muscle.
Clients who are swaybacked or feel back pain in this position generally need a pillow under the neck for support.
A variation is for the client to put the opposite foot on the therapist's shoulder *(see photo below.)* Clients should be instructed to do this as an unassisted self-stretch by letting the leg to be stretched hang off the edge of a bed.

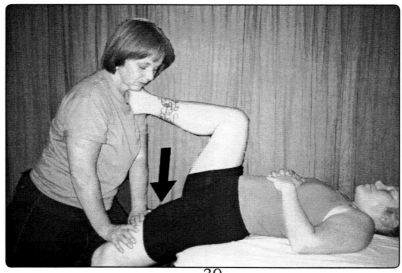

11B. ILIOPSOAS AND THIGH FLEXOR STRETCH SIDE-LYING:

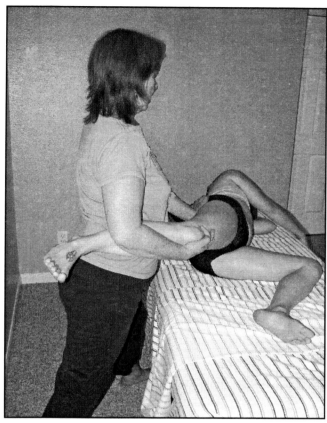

For some clients and/or therapists, this side-lying stretch may be more appropriate.

Client is side-lying on the *opposite* side of the one you want to stretch.

Step one: Ask your client to bend her knee and flex the thigh of the *bottom* leg to stabilize the pelvis.

Step two: Extend the top leg as far back as comfortably possible to lengthen the iliopsoas and secondary thigh flexors. You may wrap the leg around your waist to help hold the weight of the leg. Your uphill hand should be pushing up on the ishium as your other hand pulls the top leg back into thigh extension.

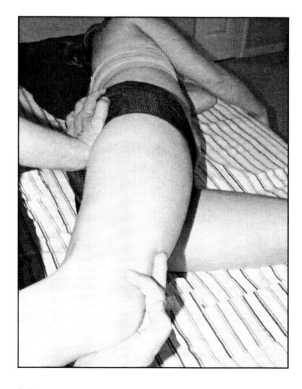

SHOULDER

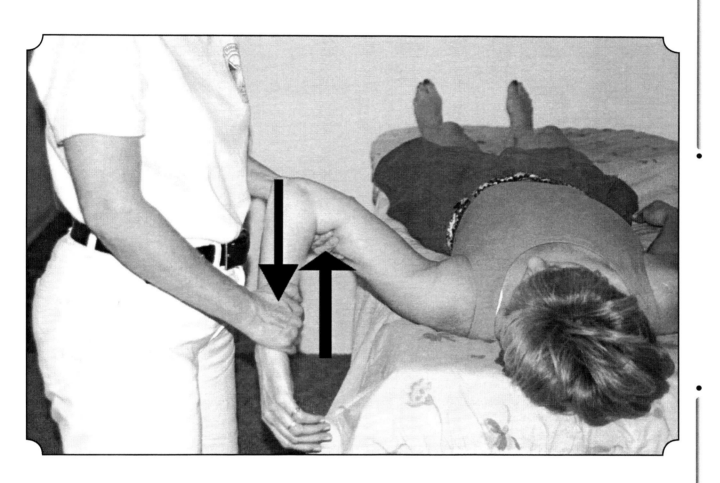

STRETCHES

SHOULDER

Subscapularis: internal (medial) rotation and adduction of the humerus. As part of the rotator cuff it helps to secure the head of the humerus in the glenoid fossa.

Supraspinatus: abduction of the humerus. As part of the rotator cuff it helps to secure the head of the humerus in the glenoid fossa.

Latissimus Dorsi and Teres Major: extension, adduction, and internal (medial) rotation of the humerus.

Rhomboids: retraction and downward rotation of the scapula.

Serratus Anterior: protraction and upward rotation of the scapula.

1. SUBSCAPULARIS STRETCH:

This muscle is usually locked short on most people, therefore stretching it along with the pectoralis major will help counteract a slumped, forward-shoulder posture.

It's often necessary to release the muscle/tendon unit of subscap's antagonists, infraspinatus and teres minor, before doing this stretch because these eccentrically overloaded and locked long muscles fight against the subscap stretch. Make sure your client is feeling the stretch in the subscapularis or pectoralis major and latissimus dorsi/teres major which are other internal rotators of the humerus.

You can release the muscle/tendon unit of infraspinatus and teres minor by sliding your hand under your client's shoulder. The tendons of infraspinatus and teres minor are under posterior deltoid. Do some gentle circular massage on posterior deltoid to muscle swim to the deeper layer where the tendons of infraspinatus and teres minor live. Once you feel that tissue soften, slide your hand medially to warm up the belly of infraspinatus and teres minor. You may need to do this several times to get what I call a "clean stretch" - meaning that the sensation of stretch is felt in subscap or pectoralis major and latissimus dorsi/teres major. I highly recommend you use PNF (antagonist and agonist contract) techniques with this perennially locked short muscle.

A. Client is supine. With client's elbow bent, abduct the humerus to 90 degrees, traction and externally rotate the humerus with your downhill hand. Gently push down on the forearm with your uphill hand and slowly increase the external rotation on the humerus with your downhill hand, maintaining the traction. Hold for 15-30 seconds.

B. As the muscle releases, move the humerus towards the head to get different fibers of subscap.

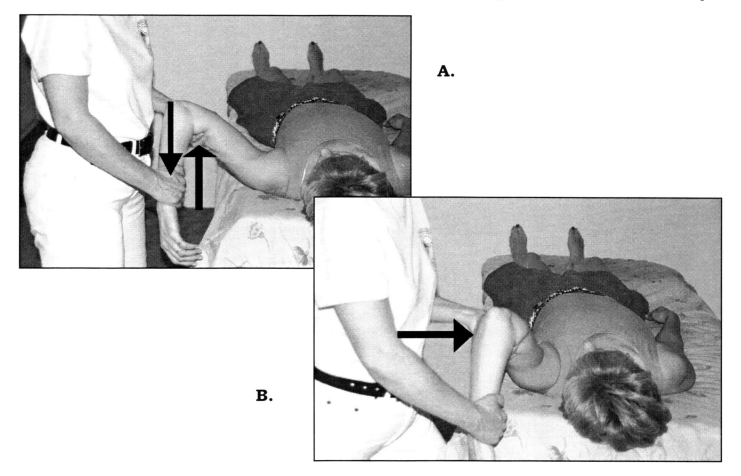

2. SUPRASPINATUS STRETCH:
Client is side-lying with a pillow under her head.

A. Your uphill hand tractions the humerus towards the client's hips while the your downhill hand presses the humerus behind the back in adduction.

B. It's helpful to pin the supraspinatus with your fingers during the stretch, as shown in photo B, to aid the client in feeling the stretch in the small supraspinatus.

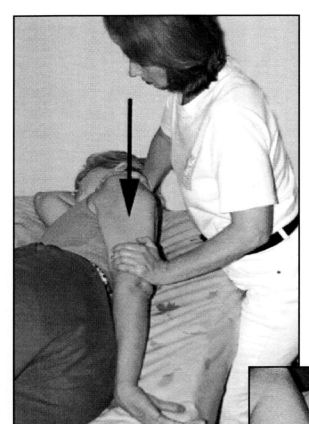

A.

B.

3. SERRATUS ANTERIOR STRETCH:

Client is side-lying on the side opposite of the one to be stretched. Press client's shoulder blade into full retraction (adduction). Experiment with downward rotation of the scapula since serratus upwardly rotates it. This is a subtle stretch, but clients with a tight serratus will find it quite pleasant.

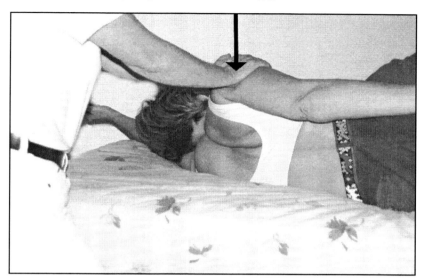

4. LATISSIMUS DORSI AND TERES MAJOR STRETCH:

Client is side-lying on the side opposite of the one to be stretched.
Step 1: The therapist abducts the arm to just behind the head. If the client finds it painful to bring the arm behind the head, which requires a large degree of external rotation of the humerus, allow the arm to rest where it's comfortable.

Step 2: Press the humerus down toward the table while gently pulling the humerus away from the hip in a tractioning move.

Step 3: Use your other hand to stabilize the torso and push the iliac crest away from the ribs.

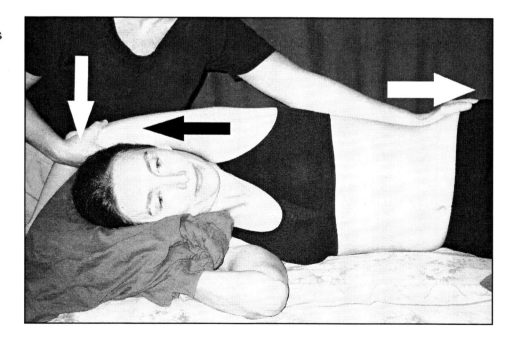

5. GENERAL STRETCH FOR TORSO, SHOULDERS, AND CHEST:

Client is supine. Ask the client to place her hands around your waist and

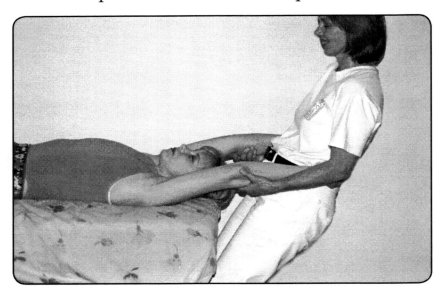

hold on. Grasp the client's humerus (not the wrist) just above both elbows and tilt back. Hold for 15-30 seconds, then lean right, then left, holding each direction for 15-30 seconds. If slippery lubricant is a problem use small towels around your hands.

A variation on this stretch is for the client to hold onto the therapist's upper arms, which includes the *lower back* in the stretch. Make sure to bend your knees, and watch for any lower back discomfort in yourself or your client.

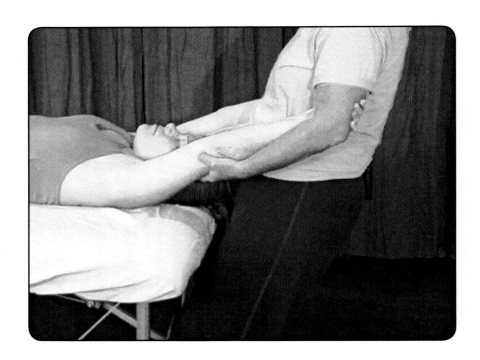

{Reminder: Take the muscle(s) slightly beyond the natural end point of the range of motion into the "stretch zone".}

6. RHOMBOID STRETCH:

The rhomboids tend to be overstretched on most people and generally need strengthening, so use this stretch sparingly. You can stretch the rhomboids from most any position. I like this supine version because it offers more control.

Slide your downhill hand under your clients' scapula, hooking the medial edge with your fingers. Grasp your clients' elbow with your uphill hand. Using both hands protract (pull the scapula away from the spine) the scapula. Instruct your client to stay flat on the table; her inclination will be to roll towards you. Hold for 15-20 seconds.

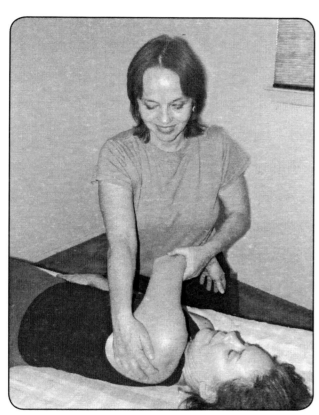

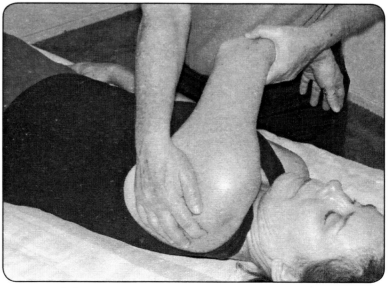

CHEST & ABDOMINAL

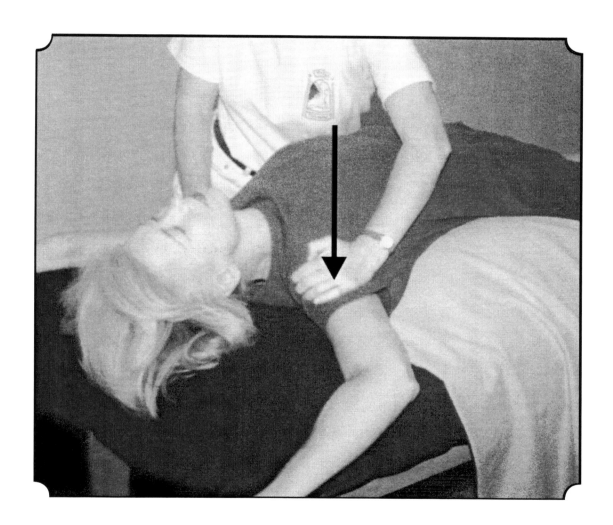

STRETCHES

CHEST

Pectoralis Major: all fibers adduct and internally rotate the humerus. Lower fibers contribute to extension while the upper fibers contribute to flexion of the humerus.

Pectoralis Minor: depresses and protracts the scapula.

ABDOMINALS

Rectus Abdominus: prime mover for spinal flexion; compresses the abdominal cavity.

External Obliques: rotates torso to opposite side; assists in spinal flexion; compresses the abdominal cavity.

Internal Obliques: rotates torso to same side; assists in spinal flexion; compresses the abdominal cavity; acts as an antagonist to the diaphragm, helping to reduce the volume of the thoracic cavity during exhalation.

1. PECTORALIS MAJOR STRETCH SUPINE:

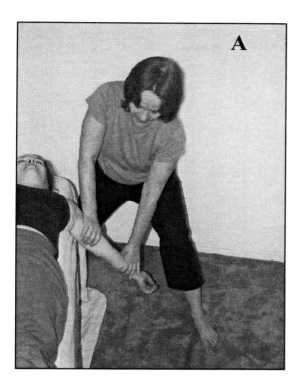

This stretches the three divisions of pectoralis major: clavicular, sternal, and costal.

A. Client is supine. Have client move close to the side of the table of the arm to be stretched. Abduct the arm to about 90° and externally (laterally) rotate the humerus. Traction the humerus. Gently press the humerus and forearm down.
*To make the stretch less intense, or if your client feels pain, tingling, or numbness in the forearm, press **only** on the humerus, not the forearm, and bend the elbow.*

B. Abduct the arm slightly higher, maintaining the external rotation and traction, and press down again.

C. Repeat this (abducting the arm slightly higher and higher, pressing down and holding) until you've reached the client's end range of motion.

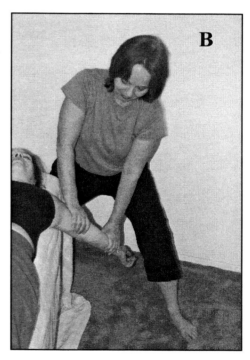

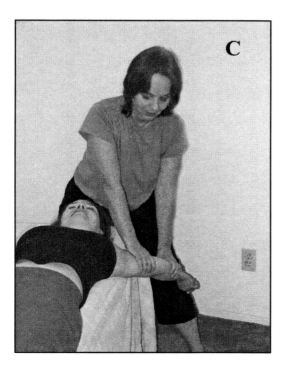

2. PECTORALIS MAJOR STRETCH PRONE:

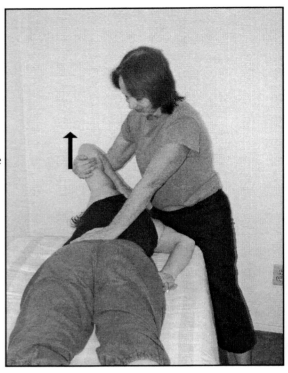

Client is prone. Stand at the head of the table. Abduct and externally rotate the humerus with the elbow bent. Place the client's hand on her head. Gently pull the elbow up towards the ceiling. Stabilize the client's pelvis with your other hand. This is easily integrated into a prone back sequence.

3. PECTORALIS MAJOR AND MINOR STRETCH:

Client is supine. Prop one or two pillows under the client's mid-back so the cervical and thoracic spine is in hyperextension and supported by the table. The number of pillows depends on the flexibility of your client. For a client with limited flexibility, start with one pillow then build up. Make sure the shoulders are externally rotated. Gently press the shoulders down towards the table. This stretch is also great for deepening the breath. The client will also be getting a gentle sternocleidomastoid stretch. You can massage the lower body while the client enjoys this stretch. Clients should be instructed to do this as an unassisted self-stretch.

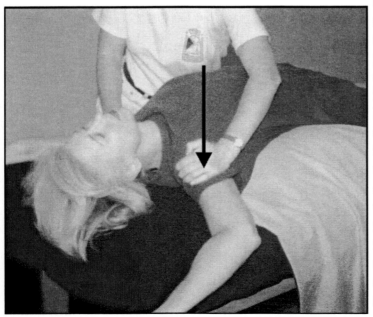

4. PECTORALIS MINOR STRETCH:

This is a more precise stretch for pec minor. Since pec minor depresses and protracts the scapula, we'll elevate and retract the scapula to stretch this often locked short muscle which can wreak havoc on our shoulders and neck.

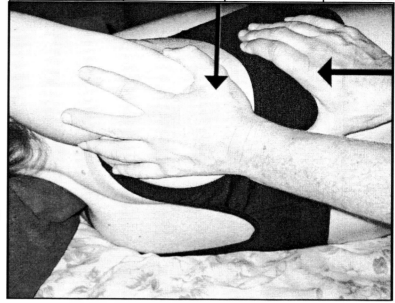

Client is side-lying with a pillow supporting the head.
Step 1: abduct the humerus to 180°.
Step 2: externally rotate the shoulder joint,
Step 3: elevate and retract (adduct) the scapula.
The arrow pointing *down* refers to the retraction of the scapula. The arrow pointing *left* refers to the elevation of the scapula. Make sure the client's lower back does not fall backward or forward.

5. ABDOMINALS AND PECTORALIS MAJOR (COBRA STRETCH):

I often do this stretch in sequence with the Cat Stretch and the Pose of Child stretch shown in the Low Back & Hip Stretches section.

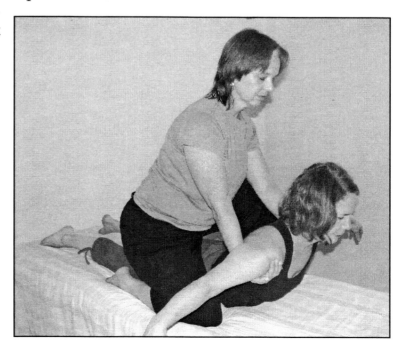

To prevent compression and discomfort in the lumbar spine, ask your client to slightly tuck her tail bone under.
Place your hands under her armpits, so that they can grasp the front of your client's shoulders. Gently and slowly, raise the client's chest off the table. Instruct her to keep her neck in alignment with the spine as most people will automatically raise the chin and hyperextend the neck.

6. OBLIQUES AND ROTATORES (UPPER BODY TWIST STRETCH):

This is a delightful and nurturing stretch that's easily integrated into a relaxation massage. You'll be able to hold the top sheet in place with the hand that's pulling your client toward you.

From across the table, slide your uphill hand under your client's back while stabilizing the pelvis with your downhill hand. Gently roll your client toward you. Notice that the therapists' hand is on the thoracic spine, not on the scapula. If it were on the scapula, this would also stretch the rhomboids and middle trapezius. Since these scapula retractors are usually over-stretched on most people, I recommend rotating the torso from the spine and not the scapula, as shown in photo right.

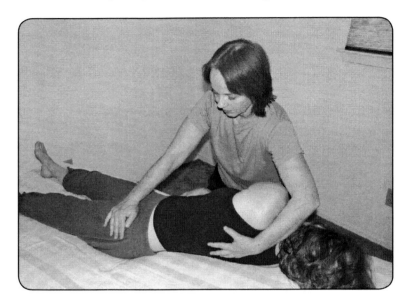

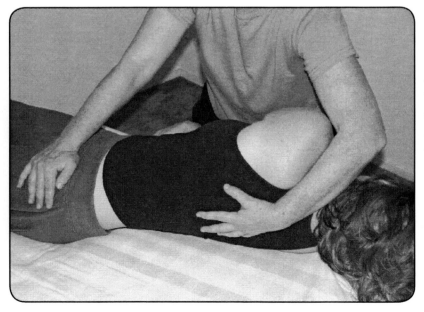

Close-up of upper body twist. By rotating the client to the right, the left internal obliques, the right external obliques and the right rotatores are being stretched.

HUMERUS & FOREARM

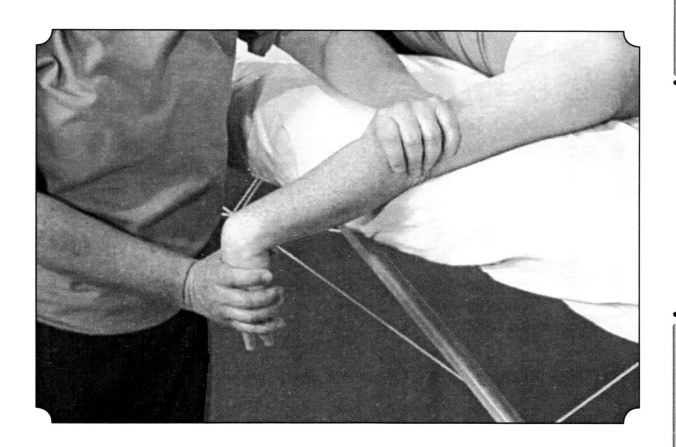

STRETCHES

HUMERUS AND FOREARMS

Biceps: flexes the elbow and supinates the forearm.

Triceps: extends the elbow; assists in adduction and extension of the shoulder joint.

Wrist Flexors *(flexor carpi radialis, flexor carpi ulnaris, palmaris longus, and flexor digitorum superficialis)*: flex, abduct, and adduct the wrist.

Wrist Extensors *(extensor carpi radialis longus and brevis, extensor carpi ulnaris and extensor digitorum)*: extend, abduct, and adduct the wrist.

1. BICEPS STRETCH:

Step 1: Client is sitting. Abduct the humerus to 90° and swing it backwards with the shoulder joint externally (laterally) rotated. The elbow must be extended and the wrist pronated (facing the floor.)

Step 2: Firmly grasp the elbow from underneath and gently pull the humerus farther back. Your client may want to twist her torso towards the arm being stretched; instruct her to twist slightly to the opposite side.

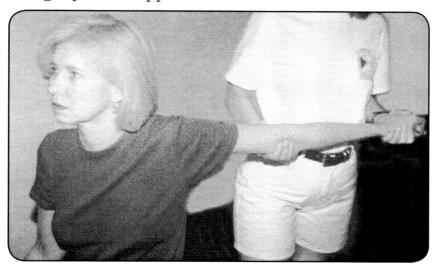

2. TRICEPS STRETCH:

Client is supine. Flex the humerus and the elbow and place the client's hand under the shoulder, palm to shoulder. Gently press down on the humerus.

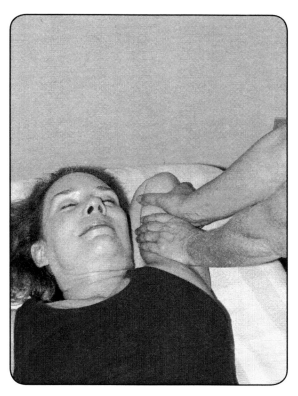

{Reminder: The sensation of stretch should be felt in the belly of the muscle and not in the tendon.}

3. WRIST FLEXORS STRETCH (flexor carpi radialis, flexor carpi ulnaris, palmaris longus, and flexor digitorum superficialis):

Client is supine. Move the wrist to be stretched off the table and turn the palm up. With your uphill hand on top of the elbow to keep it extended and stable, gently press down on the palm and fingers of her hand, hyperextending the client's wrist. Hold for 15-30 seconds.

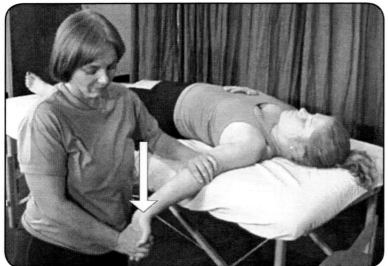

Maintaining wrist hyperextension, add various degrees of wrist abduction and adduction, (shown below), while pressing down on the palm and fingers.

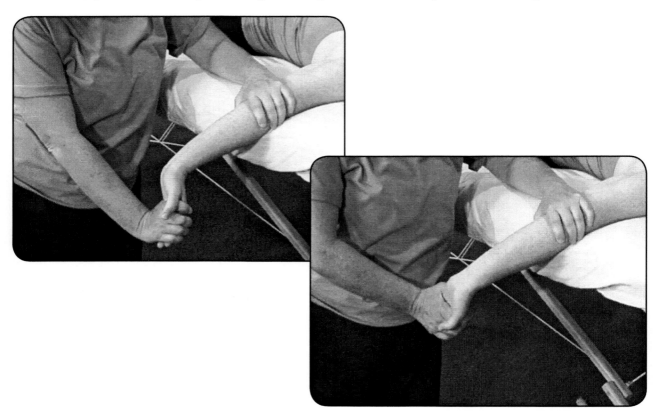

Be cautious doing this stretch on clients with carpal tunnel or other wrist problems.

4. WRIST EXTENSORS STRETCH (extensor carpi radialis longus and brevis, extensor carpi ulnaris, extensor digitorum):

Client is supine. Move the wrist to be stretched off the table and turn the palm down. With your uphill hand on top of the elbow to keep it stable and extended, gently press down on the dorsal side of the hand, flexing the wrist. Hold for 15-30 seconds.

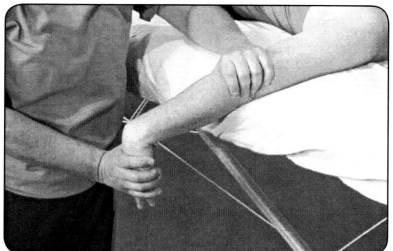

Maintaining wrist flexion, add various degrees of wrist abduction and adduction, (shown below), while pressing down on the dorsal side of the hand.

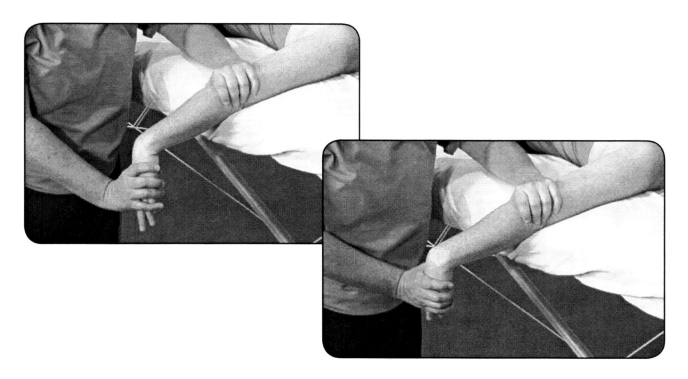

Be cautious doing this stretch on clients with carpal tunnel or other wrist problems.

THIGH & CALF

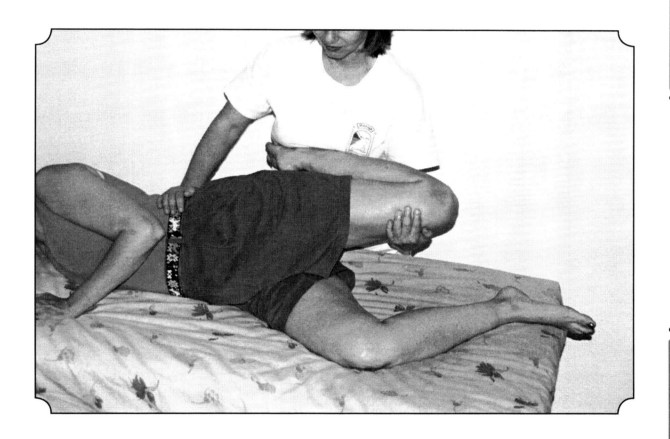

STRETCHES

THIGH

Quadriceps (*vastus medialis, intermedius, and lateralis, rectus femoris*): (all) extend the knee. Rectus femoris assists in thigh flexion.

Hamstrings (*semitendinosus, semimembranosus, and biceps femoris*): bend the knee and extend the hip.

Adductor Group (*pectineus, gracilis, adductor longus, brevis and magnus*) : all adduct the thigh. Pectineus and adductors longus and brevis, and magnus assist in thigh flexion and medial rotation. The gracilis assists in knee flexion.

CALF

Tibialis Anterior: dorsi flexes the ankle and inverts the foot.

Gastrocnemius: plantar flexes the ankle and assists in knee flexion.

Soleus: plantar flexes the ankle.

Peroneus: everts and plantar flexes the ankle.

Tibialis Posterior: inverts the foot and assists in plantar flexion; key stabilizing muscle of the lower leg.

1. QUADRICEPS STRETCH (RECTUS FEMORIS, VASTUS INTERMEDIUS, VASTUS MEDIALIS, VASTUS LATERALIS) : ★

Client is side-lying. Using this position instead of the prone position eliminates stress on the lumbar spine. Clients should also be instructed to do these as unassisted self-stretches by grasping the heel of the leg to be stretched and pressing it towards the sit bone. In the following three photographs the knee is placed at different angles. Placing the knee at different angles stretches different parts of the quads. For certain dysfunctions such as patella tracking syndrome, it's important to be able to isolate the quad stretches. For example, in patella tracking syndrome, usually the vastus lateralis is locked short while the vastus medialis is locked long. In that situation, you would concentrate on stretching the vastus lateralis and strengthening the vastus medialis.

A. RECTUS FEMORIS/VASTUS INTERMEDIUS STRETCH:

Since rectus femoris also contributes to hip flexion, hyperextend the femur by guiding the client's knee behind the pelvis and gently press the heel towards the sit bone with your torso. The therapist's right hand is stabilizing the torso, preventing hyperextension of the spine.

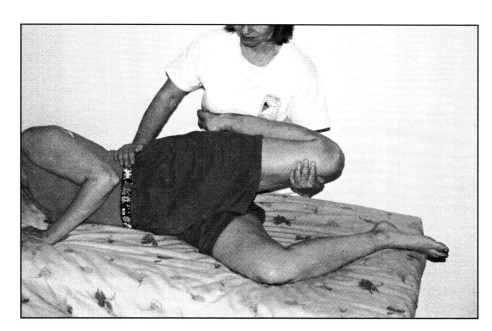

B. VASTUS MEDIALIS STRETCH: ★

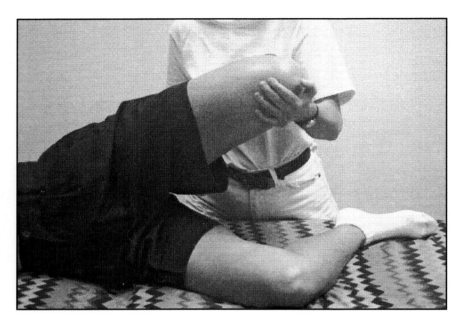

Angle client's knee toward ceiling and gently press the heel towards the sit bone. Make sure client's pelvis is in a neutral position.

C. VASTUS LATERALIS STRETCH: ★

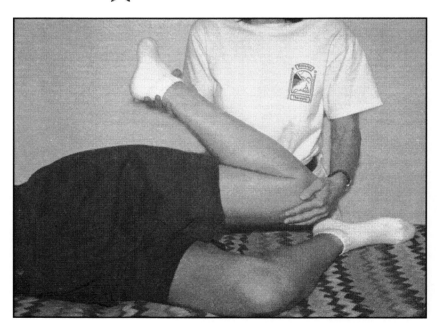

Angle client's knee towards table and gently press the heel toward the sit bone.

{Reminder: Stretching should be slow, gentle, steady and pleasurable.}

2. HAMSTRING STRETCH:

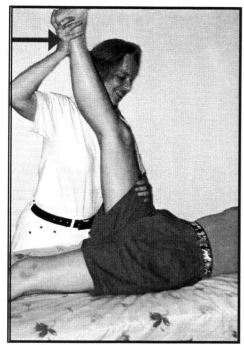

Client is supine. Extend the leg to be stretched up towards the ceiling. With one hand grasp the ankle of the leg to be stretched and gently push the leg back towards client's head. Keep the knee as straight as possible and make sure the pelvis stays on the supporting surface. It is a common mistake to allow the sit bone to come off the supporting surface, but since the hamstring attaches at the sit bone, lifting it up will negate the stretch. You can angle the leg medially and laterally to get a more specific stretch on the individual hamstring muscles. Clients should be instructed to do this as an unassisted self-stretch.

3. ADDUCTOR GROUP STRETCH:

Client is supine. Therapist can be standing on either the inside or outside of the leg to be stretched. Grasp client's leg at ankle or knee and place your other hand on the opposite iliac crest or thigh to stabilize the pelvis. Abduct the leg, keeping the clients' knee pointed towards the ceiling. **A.** Angling the leg down to the floor stretches the ***pectineus, adductor longus*** and ***brevis***. **B.** Angling the leg up towards the ceiling stretches the ***gracilis*** and ***adductor magnus***.

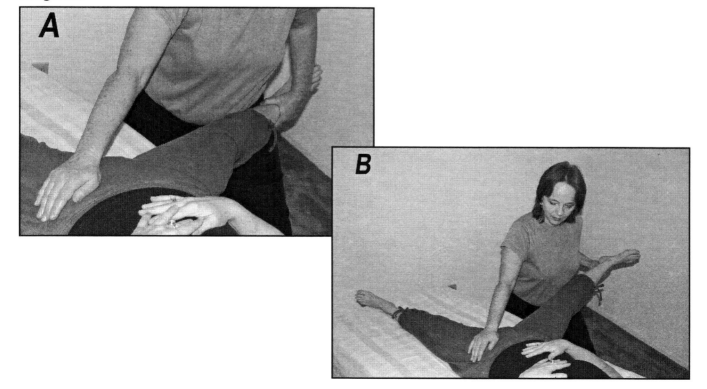

4. TIBIALIS ANTERIOR STRETCH:

This muscle is often weak and overstretched whereas the gastrocnemius and soleus are tight and need stretching, so exercise caution when deciding to stretch it. Have the client scoot down on the table so the ankle clears the table. Plantar flex (toes down) the ankle while everting (sole of the foot towards the outside) the foot. Stabilize the client's leg and foot during the stretch.

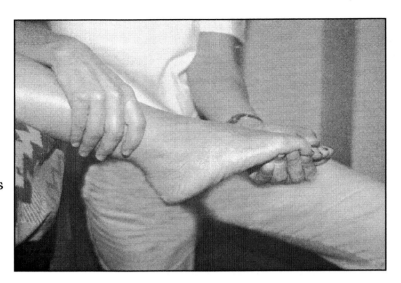

5. GASTROCNEMIUS STRETCH:

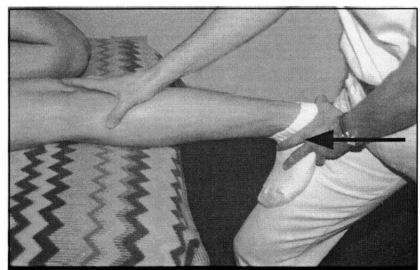

Client is prone. Have client slide down on the table so the ankle clears the table. With the client's foot against your leg or hip, use your body weight to push the bottom of the foot towards the table. Stabilize the client's leg and foot during the stretch.

{Reminder: Know the actions and attachments of the muscle you are stretching. A strong foundational knowledge of anatomy is indispensable for intelligent, intuitive bodywork.}

6. SOLEUS STRETCH:

Client is prone. Bend (flex) the knee of the leg to be stretched and press the bottom of the foot and the toes down toward the table into dorsi flexion. Stabilize the client's leg and foot during the stretch.

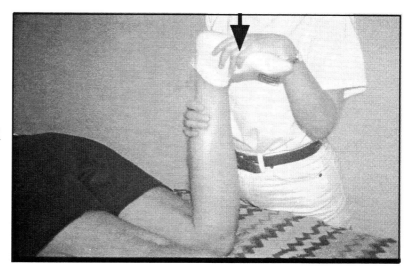

7. PERONEUS STRETCH:

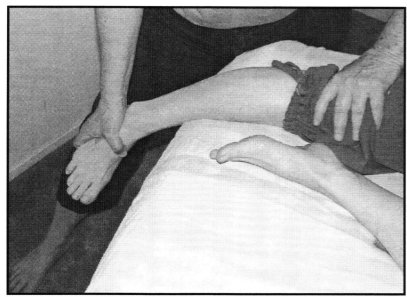

Client is side-lying. Since the peroneus muscle everts the foot, (lifts the outside of the foot off the ground), invert the foot by pressing the outside of the foot toward the floor and traction the ankle. Stabilize the client's knee during the stretch.

8. TIBIALIS POSTERIOR STRETCH:

Client is prone. Since the tibialis posterior muscle inverts the foot, (lifts the inside of the foot off the ground), and assists in plantar flexion, evert the foot by pressing the inside of the foot toward the opposite side (the lateral side of the foot) while dorsi flexing the foot. Remember to traction the ankle.

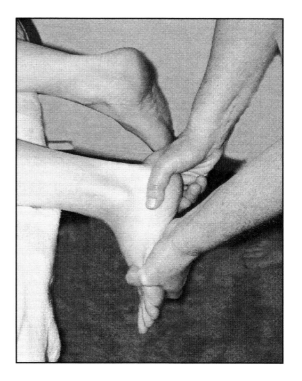

GLOSSARY

Acute: the first 24-48 hours after an injury.
Subacute: the initial inflammation and pain have subsided.
Chronic: a long-term or recurring condition.
Agonist: the prime mover.
Antagonist: the muscle that does the opposite action of the prime mover or agonist.
Check-Reining: a phenomenon in which the muscle is preventing the body from succumbing to the force of gravity.
Concentric contraction: a shortening contraction. When a muscle's attachments (origin and insertion) are brought closer together, causing a shortening of the muscle. A muscle's action (example - biceps flex the elbow) is its concentric contraction.
Eccentric contraction: a lengthening contraction. For example, if you were standing in anatomical position with your elbows bent and you straightened your elbows gravity would be doing the work, not the triceps. The triceps only extend (straighten) the elbow *against gravity*. But if you *slowly* straightened your elbows in anatomical position, your biceps would be doing an *eccentric* (lengthening) contraction.
Proprioceptors: sensory receptors located in all the movable parts of the body. They are like the internal eyes of the body that let us know where we are in space.
Synergist: a helper muscle to the prime mover.

Movement Definitions

Abduction: Lifting a body part away from the midline.
Adduction: Returning a body part to the midline.
Circumduction: Range of movements that create a complete circle (only in ball and socket joints.)
Depression: Lowering a body part (lowering the jaw.)
Dorsal Flexion: Bending the ankle so that the toes are raised.
Elevation: Lifting a body part (shoulder shrugs.)
Eversion: Turning of the sole of the foot laterally (lifting the lateral edge of the foot.)
Extension: Increasing joint angle (straightening elbows.)
Flexion: Narrowing joint angle (bending elbow.)
Hyperextension: Increasing angle more than in natural position, e.g. bending backwards.
Inversion: Turning of the sole of the foot medially (lifting the medial edge of the foot.)
Lateral flexion: Bending body sideways.
Plantar Flexion: Bending the ankle joint so toes point downwards.
Pronation: Internal rotation of the radius resulting in a palm down position of the hand.
Protraction: Moving a body part outwards, e.g. moving the scapulae away from the spine.
Pronation: External rotation of the radius resulting in a palm up position of the hand.**Retraction:** Bringing a body part back, e.g. moving the scapulae toward the spine.
Rotation: Turning a body part on axis (not rotation all the way round - see circumduction.)

Joint Movements

ANKLE & FOOT: dorsi flexion, plantar flexion, inversion, eversion, abduction, adduction.

ELBOW: flexion, extension.

JAW: depression, elevation, protraction, retraction, lateral deviation (moving the jaw side to side.)

KNEE: flexion, extension, hyperextension, internal and external rotation.

SHOULDER GIRDLE (scapula and clavicle): elevation, depression, retraction (adduction), protraction (abduction), upward rotation, downward rotation.

SHOULDER JOINT (humerus): abduction, adduction, flexion, extension, internal rotation, external rotation, circumduction.

SPINE: flexion, extension, hyperextension, lateral flexion, rotation.

THIGH (hip): abduction, adduction, flexion, extension, internal rotation, external rotation, circumduction.

WRISTS: abduction, adduction, flexion, extension.

SUGGESTED READING

Anderson, Bob: **Stretching**, Shelter Publications.
Benjamen, Ben: **Are You Tense?**, Pantheon Books.
Carrico, Maria: **Yoga Journal's Yoga Basics**, Henry Holt & Co.
Dixon, Marian Wolfe: **Body Mechanics and Self Care Manual,** Prentice Hall.
Mattes, Aaron: **Active Isolated Stretching**, self-published.
Sweigard, Lulu: **Human Movement Potential - Its Ideokinetic Facilitation**, Harper and Row.
Travell, Janet & Simons, David: **Myofascial Pain and Dysfunction: The Trigger Point Manual**, William and Wilkens.

"It's what you learn after you know it all that counts."
-John Wooden

Index

A

ABDOMINALS/PEC MAJOR STRETCH 43
ABDUCTOR STRETCH 28
ACTIVE RESISTIVE STRETCHES 4
ACUTE 8
ADDUCTOR GROUP STRETCH 54
ADDUCTOR LONGUS, BREVIS AND MAGNUS ACTIONS 51
AGONIST 57
ANTAGONIST 57
ANTAGONIST-CONTRACTION 4

B

BICEPS ACTIONS 46
BICEPS STRETCH 47
BODY MECHANICS 9

C

CAT STRETCH 23
CHECK-REIGNING 3
CHRONIC INJURIES 57
COBRA STRETCH 43
CONCENTRIC 57

E

ECCENTRIC 3, 57
ERECTOR SPINAE ACTIONS 18
ERECTOR SPINAE STRETCHES 19
EXTERNAL OBLIQUES ACTIONS 40

F

FIRST-DEGREE MUSCLE STRAIN 8

G

GASTROCNEMIUS 51, 55
GLOSSARY 57
GLUTEUS MAXIMUS ACTIONS 18
GLUTEUS MAXIMUS STRETCH 19
GLUTEUS MINIMUS/MEDIUS ACTIONS 18
GLUTEUS MINIMUS/MEDIUS STRETCHES 27, 28
GRACILIS ACTIONS 51
GRACILIS STRETCH 54
GUIDELINES FOR STRETCHING 6

H

HAMSTRINGS ACTIONS 51
HAMSTRING STRETCH 54

I

ILIOPSOAS ACTIONS 18
ILIOPSOAS STRETCH 30, 31
INTERNAL OBLIQUES ACTIONS 40

J

JOINT MOVEMENTS 58

L

LATISSIMUS DORSI ACTIONS 33
LATISSIMUS DORSI STRETCH 36
LORDOSIS 3

M

MASSETER ACTIONS 11
MASSETER STRETCH 16
MOVEMENT DEFINITIONS 57
MULTIFIDI ACTIONS 18
MULTIFIDI STRETCHES 22, 23, 24

O

OBLIQUES STRETCH 44
OVER-STRETCHING 3

P

PASSIVE STRETCHING 4
PECTINEUS ACTIONS 51
PECTINEUS STRETCH 54
PECTORALIS MAJOR ACTIONS 40
PECTORALIS MAJOR STRETCH 41, 42
PECTORALIS MINOR ACTIONS 40
PECTORALIS MINOR STRETCH 43
PERONEUS ACTIONS 51
PERONEUS STRETCH 56
PHYSIOLOGICAL BARRIER 6
PIRIFORMIS ACTIONS 18
PIRIFORMIS STRETCH 29
POSE OF CHILD STRETCH 24
POST INJURY STRETCHING 8

Q

QUADRATUS LUMBORUM ACTIONS 18
QUADRATUS LUMBORUM STRETCHES 26, 27, 28
QUADRICEPS ACTIONS 51
QUADRICEPS STRETCH 52

R

RECTUS ABDOMINUS ACTIONS 40
RECTUS FEMORIS STRETCH 52
RHOMBOIDS ACTIONS 33
RHOMBOID STRETCH 38
ROTATORES ACTIONS 18
ROTATORES STRETCHES 22, 44

S

SCALENES ACTIONS 11

Scalenes stretch 14
second-degree muscle strain 8
Serratus Anterior actions 33
Serratus anterior stretch 36
Soleus actions 51
Soleus stretch 56
Sternocleidomastoid actions 11
Sternocleidomastoid stretch 15
stretch reflex 3, 6
sub-acute 8
Subscapularis actions 33
Subscapularis stretch 34
Suggested Reading 58
Supraspinatus actions 33
Supraspinatus stretch 35

T

temporalis muscle 11, 16
Tensor fasciae latae actions 18
Tensor fasciae latae stretches 26, 27
Teres Major actions 33
Teres major stretch 36
third-degree muscle strain 8
tibialis anterior actions 51
tibialis anterior stretch 55
Tibialis Posterior actions 51
Trapezius actions 11
Trapezius stretch 14
Tricep actions 46
Triceps stretch 47
Types of stretching 4

U

upper body twist stretch 44

V

Vastus Intermedius stretch 52
Vastus Lateralis stretch 53
Vastus Medialis Stretch 53

W

Wrist Extensors 46, 49
Wrist Flexors 46, 48

ABOUT THE AUTHOR

Peggy Lamb, MA, LMT, NCTMB, has been practicing massage since 1986 and is also the author of ***Releasing The Rotator Cuff***. She received her initial training at the New Mexico Academy of Massage and Advanced Healing Arts in Santa Fe and Wellness Skills, Inc., in Dallas. She taught Clinical Anatomy and Physiology, Trigger Point Therapy and Swedish Technique at Wellness Skills, Inc. for nine years and was on the faculty of Texas Healing Arts Institute in Austin for four years. In addition to her extensive training in massage therapy, Peggy holds a Masters Degree in Dance from American University in Washington, D.C. She also teaches dance and yoga and is a personal trainer. Peggy is available for ***"Stretch Your Clients"*** workshops and can be reached at **(512) 833-0179** or email **info@massagepublications.com**.

Other relevant workshops that Peggy is available to teach are ***"Releasing The Rotator Cuff"*** and ***"Tips and Tricks for the Lower Back: Releasing the Iliopsoas and Quadratus Lumborum"***. She brings her eclectic and extensive background into her teaching for an interesting, fun, and enlightening learning experience. A full listing of Peggy's Continuing Education workshops approved by the Texas Department of Health, Florida Department of Health, AMTA, ABMP, and NCBTMB can be found at: **www.massagepublications.com**.

Bring joy, ease suffering and create beauty, then dance like you mean it!

CD-ROM AGREEMENT AND DISCLAIMER

Please read the following carefully before using the CD-ROM:

DISCLAIMER
This software is sold as is without warranty of any kind, either expressed or implied, including but not limited to the implied warranties of merchantability and fitness for a particular purpose. Neither the author (Peggy Lamb, MA; RMT) nor the publisher (Massage Publications) nor its dealers or distributors assumes any liability for any alleged or actual damages arising from the use of this CD-ROM. In no event will the author (Peggy Lamb, MA; RMT) nor the publisher (Massage Publications) be liable to you for any damages, including any loss of profit or other incidental, special or consequential damages even if the author (Peggy Lamb, MA; RMT) or the publisher (Massage Publications) has been advised of the possibility of such damages. Some states do not allow the exclusion of implied warranties, so the exclusion may not apply to you.

LICENSE
You are licensed to use the CD-ROM copyrighted by the author on a single computer. You may make one copy of the software for back-up purpose only. Making copies of the software for any other purposes is a violation of the United States copyright laws.

If you have questions about this agreement please contact the author at: info@massagepublications.com.

Systems requirements: PC with Windows 95 ,98, XP, 2000, Vista and Windows 7; a CD-ROM drive; 100MHz or faster Pentium or compatible processor; 32 MB of available RAM; 800x600 resolution and 16 bit color. *This CD-ROM is not compatible with Macintosh computers.*

If you have AutoPlay enabled, insert the CD-ROM into your CD drive. If you have AutoPlay *disabled* on your computer the CD-ROM will not automatically run. To open the program manually, double click on My Computer on your desktop, double click on your CD-ROM drive, then double click the **StretchYourClients.exe** file.